MASTERING
HEALTHY EATING

Your Guide to Achieving

Nutritional Excellence

COPYRIGHT OWNER

TABLE OF CONTENTS

CHAPTER 1: SIMPLIFYING NUTRITION FOR HEALTH AND WELL-BEING

CHAPTER 2: WHY HEALTHY EATING IMPORTANT?

CHAPTER 3: UNDERSTANDING YOUR CONNECTION WITH FOOD

CHAPTER 4: THE PERIL OF EAT LESS PATTERNS

CHAPTER 5: THE FOOD GUIDELINES

CHAPTER 6: FOOD AS MEDICINE:A GUIDE TO A HEALTHY LIFE

CHAPTER 7: EATING VEGETABLES IS GOOD

CHAPTER 8: EATING FRUITS NOURISH OUR BODY

CHAPTER 9: THE HEALTH BENEFIT OF MEAT

INTRODUCTION

Food is an essential aspect of human life, but in today's modern world Nowadays, it is becoming more and more complicated. With countless food trends, conflicting nutrition advice, and convenient but often unhealthy food options, many people have difficulty effectively navigating the field of nutrition. This introduction aims to explore a simple approach to eating that prioritizes simplicity, balance, and conscious consumption.
Eating food is a common phenomenon in the world that allows humanity to grow and live healthily. It is very important to combine a variety of suitable foods to benefit the human body. It is also a challenge in life.
For many reasons, one of the most difficult things for people is to eat well. Whether it's because we have limited access to resources in all areas or because we often have access to poor diets, there are many reasons why healthy eating can help, is a challenge.

There is no doubt that eating almost anything is possible and it will feed us. We will continue at any time and can consider ourselves solid. But is it good to eat less processed foods and sugary drinks? Just because we are alive doesn't mean we are healthy. And the more experience we gain, the more our terrible tendencies begin to catch up with us.

It is extremely important to adopt healthy eating habits from an early age, or at least as early as possible, to prevent problems from arising in the future. You don't want to wake up one day and realize that you've been malnourished for years and it's causing almost irreversible complications. We all need to be more responsible with what we put into our bodies because otherwise, it can become extremely dangerous.

Of course, as we get older and have If you can go back to your mistakes, . We realize that there were things we could have done and should have done but we didn't because we weren't aware of the harm or were simply lazy. Just having simple knowledge does not necessarily make the need to do something health-conscious a reality.

It requires us to face the suffering that can arise from unhealthy choices before doing so. become more aware of how we treat our bodies and overall health. When we can't see the reality of the consequences of our actions, they can seem very distant and confusing. We can even eliminate them. This can be a very tiring place. Especially when you're dealing with the side effects of poor diet and lack of healthy eating.

Everyone deserves the chance to be the best version of themselves. Feasibility. However, if we don't even acknowledge the fact that an unhealthy diet can throw us off course, even in the present moment, then we are saying goodbye to a future as good as there can be.

But all that can change. By reading this book, you will understand the importance of healthy eating and the impact food has on our bodies and functions.
Sometimes, it's hard to get in the right direction without understanding exactly why our bodies react to food the way he does. But there are many ways to begin to understand why eating healthy foods is important and how to start your healthy eating journey. Let's not waste any more time. We should start eating healthy today

CHAPTER 1
Simplifying Nutrition for Health and Well-being

The need for simplicity in Nutrition a society saturated with information, simplicity in nutrition has become a rarity. The popularity of diets that promise quick fixes and the marketing of processed
foods often obscures the fundamentals of healthy eating. The direct approach to eating aims to eliminate this complexity, bringing clarity amid confusion.

Principles of the direct approach

1. Emphasis on whole foods: Eating whole, unprocessed foods is at the heart of a simple approach to eating. These foods, such as fruits, vegetables, whole grains, and lean proteins, provide essential nutrients without added sugar, unhealthy fats, and artificial additives.
2. Balanced macro-nutrients: Understanding the balance of macro-nutrients (carbohydrates, proteins, and fats) is important. Instead of disregarding a specific macro-nutrient, the direct approach encourages balanced intake tailored to individual needs and goals.

3. Mindful eating: Mindfulness plays a central role in our approach to eating. This involves paying attention to hunger and fullness signals, eating slowly, and enjoying the taste and texture of foods. By promoting mindful eating practices, individuals can foster a healthier relationship with food and avoid overeating.

4. Portion control: Portion sizes in modern diets have exploded, contributing to the obesity epidemic. The direct approach advocates portion control, helping individuals understand appropriate portion sizes and preventing excessive calorie intake.

5. Personalization: There is no one-size-fits-all approach to nutrition. A direct approach encourages individuals to personalize their dietary choices based on their unique nutritional needs, preferences, and health

goals.

Benefits of a Direct Approach to Eating

Improved Health Markers: Adopting a direct approach to eating can lead to improved blood sugar levels, cholesterol profiles, and overall cardiovascular health.

Weight Management: By focusing on whole foods and portion control, individuals can achieve and maintain a healthy weight more effectively than with restrictive diets.

Enhanced Energy Levels: Nutrient-dense foods provide sustained energy throughout the day, reducing the reliance on stimulants like caffeine and sugar.

Better Digestive Health: Whole foods rich in fiber promote optimal digestion and gut health, reducing the risk of gastrointestinal disorders.

Practical Tips for Implementation

1. Meal Planning: Plan meals to ensure balanced nutrition and avoid last-minute unhealthy choices.

2. Grocery Shopping: Prioritize shopping in the perimeter of grocery stores, where whole foods like fresh produce, meats, and dairy are typically located.

3. Cooking at Home: Prepare meals at home using fresh ingredients to have better control over what goes into your food.

4. Reading Labels: When purchasing packaged foods, read labels carefully to avoid items high in added sugars, unhealthy fats, and sodium.

5. Hydration: Remember that hydration is an important aspect of nutrition; drink water throughout the day to support overall health.

A simple approach to eating offers a fresh perspective on nutrition, emphasizing simplicity, balance, and conscious consumption. By focusing on whole foods, balanced macro-nutrients, portion control, and personal variety of food, individuals can achieve optimal health and wellness without the pitfalls of Modern food confusion. This introduction sets the stage for a more detailed exploration of each of these principles, providing practical information and evidence-based recommendations for taking a hands-on approach to everyday eating.

Through this approach, individuals can embark on a journey towards better health, one meal at a time.

CHAPTER 2

WHY HEALTHY EATING IMPORTANT?

Here's a comprehensive exploration of why healthy eating is important, covering various aspects such as physiological benefits, mental well-being, social and economic implications, environmental sustainability, and practical tips for adopting a healthier diet.

Healthy eating is more than just a dietary choice; it is a fundamental pillar of overall well-being and longevity. In today's fast-paced world, where convenience often trumps nutrition, understanding the profound significance of healthy eating is crucial. This essay delves deep into the multifaceted reasons why healthy eating matters, encompassing its impact on physical health, mental clarity, societal dynamics, economic outcomes, environmental sustainability, and practical strategies for adopting and maintaining a healthy diet.

Physiological Benefits of Healthy Eating

1.Nutrient Sufficiency

2.Disease Prevention

1. Nutrient Sufficiency

A diet rich in essential nutrients is fundamental for maintaining optimal health and preventing chronic diseases. Essential nutrients include vitamins, minerals, proteins, fats, and carbohydrates, each playing a crucial role in bodily functions.

1. Vitamins and Minerals: These micro-nutrients are

essential for processes such as energy production, immune function, and cell repair.

2. Protein: Necessary for building and repairing tissues, protein also plays a role in producing enzymes and hormones.

3. Fats: Healthy fats, such as omega-3 fatty acids, are essential for brain function, hormone regulation, and inflammation control.

4. Carbohydrates: are the body's main source of energy, especially important for brain function and physical activity.

2.Disease prevention
1. Heart health: A diet low in saturated fat and high in fruits, vegetables, whole grains and lean protein may reduce the risk of heart disease and stroke.

2. Diabetes management: Controlling blood sugar levels through a balanced diet helps prevent and control type 2 diabetes.

3. Cancer prevention: Certain foods rich in antioxidants and photochemical have been linked to a reduced risk of cancer.

Weight control and energy balance

1 . Calorie control: A healthy diet emphasizes portion control and choosing nutrient-rich foods, which help maintain a healthy weight.

2. Energy levels: Balanced nutrition promotes sustained energy levels throughout the day, reducing the need for quick energy boosts from sugary snacks or caffeinated beverages.

Health Intestinal health and digestive function

1. Fiber and digestion: Fiber-rich foods promote healthy digestion,

prevent constipation, and support a diverse gut micro-biome, essential for immune function and overall health.

2. Gut-brain axis: New research shows that gut health can influence mental health and regulate mood through the gut-brain axis.

Psychological and mental health Regulates mood and cognitive function

1. Brain health: Essential nutrients, such as omega-3 fatty acids, B vitamins, and antioxidants, support cognitive function, memory, and mood regulation.

2. Mental clarity: Stable blood sugar levels and adequate hydration contribute to mental clarity, concentration, and productivity.

Mental health disorders

1. Impact of diet: Research shows a link between diet quality and mental health disorders such as depression and anxiety.

2. Serotonin production: The amino acid tryptophan, found in some foods, is essential for the production of serotonin, a neurotransmitter that regulates mood and sleep.

Social Implications and Economics

Health disparities and access to healthy foods

1. Food security: Socioeconomic factors often affect access to nutritious food options, leading to disparities in health outcomes.

2. Health Care Costs: Preventing chronic disease through a healthy diet can reduce health care costs and improve overall public health.

Workplace Productivity

1. Employee Health: Healthy employee eating habits can reduce absenteeism, improve productivity, and improve workplace morale.

2. Corporate wellness programs: Many companies implement wellness programs that promote physical activity and healthy eating to improve employee health and reduce health-care costs.

Environmental sustainability

Sustainable food systems

1. Resource efficiency: Sustainable diets emphasize plant-based foods and minimize the environmental impact of food production, including water use, land use, and greenhouse gas emissions.

2. Conserving biodiversity: Supporting biodiversity through sustainable agriculture ensures resilient food systems and healthy ecosystems.

Reduce food waste

1. Consumer awareness: Educating consumers about food waste reduction strategies, such as meal planning and proper storage, can minimize the environmental impact of food waste products.

2. Circular economy: promoting a circular economy in the food system, from production to consumption to waste management, supporting environmental sustainability goals.

Words Practical advice for adopting healthy eating habits

Principles of a balanced diet

1. My Plate Template: Use visual aids like My Plate Template to guide portion sizes and food choices, focusing on fruits, vegetables, lean proteins, whole grains, and dairy.

2. Meal planning: Plan meals to ensure nutritional balance and minimize reliance on processed and takeout foods.

3. Healthy cooking techniques: Use healthy cooking methods such as grilling, steaming, or grilling instead of frying, to preserve nutrients and reduce added fat.

Eating well as a practice daily

1. Slow down: Eat slowly and mindfully, savoring each bite and paying attention to hunger and fullness signals.

2. Portion control: Use smaller plates and bowls to control portion sizes and

avoid overeating.

3. Drink water regularly: Drink plenty of water on daily basis for improvement of your healthy body

Education and Awareness

1. Read nutrition labels: Learn how to read nutrition labels to make informed choices about packaged foods and beverages.

2. Community Programs: Participate in community nutrition programs and workshops to learn about healthy eating and cooking skills.

3. Family and social support: Encourage family and friends to adopt healthy eating habits together, creating an environment for long-term success.

Healthy eating is more than just a choice of employee; it is an important determinant of personal health, social well-being, economic stability, and environmental sustainability. Individuals can benefit from improved physical and mental health by prioritizing nutrient-dense foods, controlling portion sizes, and promoting access to healthy food choices: mental health, reduced health-care costs, increased productivity, and a sustainable food future. Adopting a healthy diet as a lifestyle choice helps individuals make informed decisions that have a positive impact on their health and contribute to a healthier, happier society. than. generally happier.

A healthy diet is important for many reasons. Most of us are aware of the growing obesity epidemic in North America. This is especially true for the United States as a whole. There is even a term to describe the way many Americans eat and it is called the SAD diet.SAD stands for Standard American Diet and refers to a diet that is low in vegetables, high in fat and sugar, and lacking in nutrients. Processed foods are part of the SAD diet. These are foods that are easily available, consumed, and prepared quickly but have negative long-term health effects. If you don't want to become obese, you should avoid eating such processed foods regularly and focus on eating whole grains, fruits, vegetables, and meats that have not been treated with hormones and other chemicals that can eventually enter your body and cause problems. Unfortunately, in North America, we have so many options to skip meal prep. We have so many things at our disposal and the amount of money you have to spend on them. Poor quality food is much lower than the amount of money you would spend on good food. It may seem strange that buying organic food is more expensive than buying food that will cause health problems in the long run, but that is the law of supply and demand. In addition, processed foods are mass-produced and generate huge profits thanks to their convenience. This is why, in many ways, the obesity epidemic in North America is not surprising. Nutrition is not the first on the list of companies trying to profit from people's laziness in the kitchen. However, there are many reasons why healthy eating is important and there are good reasons to avoid processed foods and the standard American diet. For example, if you don't want to become obese, you should check out the rest of this book to find ways to improve your diet and start a healthier lifestyle. Another reason to eat If you drink healthy, you could be making yourself susceptible to disease by eating unhealthy foods and following the standard American diet that is high in fat and sugar. Diabetes can develop as a result of poor diet and can often be treated with a healthy diet. Finally, type II diabetes is a disease that can be maintained and controlled by good habits and triggered by poor eating habits. If you want to avoid these types of difficulties and complications, you must do your best to be cautious in your food choices. Other diseases can also result from poor diet. High blood pressure is common, as are other chronic diseases. Osteoporosis can affect many people later in life because they did not make healthy food choices earlier. You may suffer from poor bone health, high blood pressure, or even heart problems. All of this can be very demanding on your body and cause significant stress, which can ultimately be very dangerous.

If you want to demonstrate to your family that you care, it's important to start making choices now that will help you stay in their lives for as long as possible. Poor health doesn't just affect you - it also impacts the people around you. When they see you suffering because of bad choices, they suffer too. Do your best to make the right choices not only for yourself but for your family in the long run. This book will lead.

CHAPTER 3

UNDERSTANDING YOUR CONNECTION WITH FOOD

Understanding your relationship with food is a deeply personal and multifaceted journey, intertwined with many different aspects of your life. It goes beyond mere nutrition to include emotions, habits, culture, and even spirituality. This complex relationship affects not only your physical health but also your mental and emotional health.

At its core, food acts as fuel for the body, provides essential nutrients to maintain life, and supports body functions. However, our modern relationship with food often goes beyond nutritional needs. Many factors shape how we interact with food, including upbringing, social influences, psychological factors, and environmental cues.

An important aspect of understanding your relationship with food is recognizing the emotional component. For many people, food is associated with feelings of comfort, celebration, stress relief, or even guilt and shame. Emotional eating, whether in response to positive or negative emotions, can lead to unhealthy habits and contribute to problems such as overeating or restrictive eating.

Cultural and social influences also play an important role in shaping eating habits and attitudes toward food. Traditional dishes, family mealtime customs, and social norms related to body image all contribute to how we view and consume food. These effects can be both positive and negative, affecting our food choices and overall health.

In addition, understanding your relationship with food requires awareness of how external factors influence eating behavior. Food advertising, the availability of processed foods, and social norms around eating out can all influence what, when, and how much we eat. The food environment we live in can support or hinder our efforts to maintain a healthy relationship with food.

Another aspect to consider is the psychological aspect of eating behavior. Factors such as stress, boredom, loneliness, and self-esteem can all affect our relationship with food. Some people may use food as a coping mechanism, seeking comfort or distraction through eating, while others may suffer from disorders such as binge eating disorder or anorexia nervosa.

Spirituality and mindfulness also play a role in how we approach food. Practices like mindful eating encourage people to pay attention to their sensory experiences while eating, thereby cultivating a deeper connection with food and promoting healthier eating habits. Spiritual beliefs and dietary practices can also shape attitudes toward food, influencing choices based on ethical, environmental, or religious considerations.

Understanding and improving your relationship with food often involves developing conscious eating habits and cultivating emotional self-awareness. It may also involve seeking support from medical professionals, nutritionists, or therapists to address underlying issues and develop a healthier relationship with food.

Ultimately, the journey of understanding your relationship with food is a dynamic and ever-evolving process. It requires personal reflection, awareness of outside influences, and a commitment to promoting a balanced approach to eating. By better understanding your unique relationship with food and making informed choices, you can foster a healthier, more fulfilling relationship with food and with yourself.

Over time, people begin to form certain habits. "We develop habits in every area of our lives.". We develop hygiene habits, eating habits, work habits, and all kinds of other habits. However, they are often quite oblivious to our habits until they start affecting us negatively. And even then, when we begin to understand that our habits have little effect on us, changing them can be difficult. This is the absolute truth.

Habits are things we do almost unconsciously. We are born to follow these habits and it takes a lot of willpower to break out of that vicious cycle.

When you begin to understand that your relationship with food has a lot to do with it. With the habits and routines you have created that you can continue to shape and cultivate, it becomes much easier to change your thinking.

When you recognize the effects impact and importance of your future and make positive choices about these, it can make you better prepared to eat healthily and less likely to make choices that negatively impact your future. Very bad for you and your future.

To be honest, many of us seem to view the future as bleak. We don't see enough reason to change our habits, because if we don't think we have something good to look forward to, it doesn't matter whether we make the right choice or not. We don't know how we can prepare the future so that it is in our best interest. Maybe it's because we don't believe we have the right to decide our lives.

"If you can relate to this feeling, there's no need to worry.". This is very common in the human experience. We are often discouraged from taking control and using our power from a young age and sometimes stop believing that we have any power over our lives because others often tell us to. What to do.

As a child, this made sense."It's always the case that children know what's best for them." But this can encourage a helpless mindset that leaves us struggling to understand that the consequences of our actions can begin to shape who we are and how we express ourselves. Close to the world.

That's all. Why it's important to take steps to help you understand yourself and your eating habits. When did your habit start? How did you get this habit? For what? What benefits do you get from this habit? What negative effects are you experiencing from this habit?

Ask yourself as many of these questions as possible so you can begin to truly understand how you are shaping your future. Breed yourself by the food you are eating. Are you creating a healthy and energetic future or are you creating a future that is dark and likely to cause many negative health consequences?

Next, evaluate and Value your sense of self-discipline. Can you maintain discipline in your choices? Or is this an area where you are struggling? Discipline can be difficult for everyone, and if you have trouble maintaining discipline, you should find different ways to encourage yourself to become a more disciplined person, both physically and mentally. Both practical and spiritual aspects.

Only then will you have what it takes to start your healthy eating journey? Like it or not, unhealthy choices exist everywhere. They are easy and addictive.

If we let ourselves be influenced by these poor choices and do nothing to change our habits,
Sometimes it doesn't matter whether you eat healthy or not. The negative effects will continue to invade your body and

wait to appear when you least expect it.

In some ways, unhealthy eating is a type of self-destruction Self-sabotage that many of us suffer from. Whether it's because of low self-esteem or simply because we're unhappy with our circumstances and don't trust the future, self-destructive eating habits are dangerous. You need to look inward and value your life and your future before eating healthy.

There are many ways to do this and if possible, you can even seek advice. Mental health professional's opinion. To support. Sometimes they can help us spot biases and negative patterns in our lives that we are not always aware of. Once you understand and accept these, you can more easily overcome them and take the necessary steps to make positive choices.

Even if you seek help from a trained professional or not, you will encounter a lot of problems what can be done to change your mind? As long as you understand that you deserve a healthy body and a positive future, you will permit yourself to take the necessary steps to get there.

But if you don't feel like If you feel satisfied with yourself, it will be much more difficult. Overall, understanding yourself, your habits, your mental blocks, and your discipline will help you on your journey.

We can all take steps every day to become our best selves, and eating healthy is a big step in that direction. And that's a step we can take today!

Chapter 4

The Perils Of **Eat Less** Pattern

In a world where diets overpower highlights and social media supports, the charm of fast fixes and enthusiastic changes regularly rules the potential risks sneaking behind restrictive eating plans. From spasmodic fasting to exceptional low-calorie organizations, various people turn to these diets the intrigued of weight hardship, well-being benefits, or essentially as a suggestion for controlling their relationship with food. In any case, what begins as a well-intention effort to form strides in well-being can in a few cases wind into a hazardous cycle of physical and mental harm.

The perils of eat-less plans intensify and remove past the surface-level ensure of shedding pounds. They jump into the complexities of human physiology, brain inquiry, and social stream, shaping not because of how we see ourselves but moreover how we associate with the world around us. This introduction explores these perils in significance, highlighting the multifaceted perils related to restrictive eating and giving a comprehensive understanding of why these plans can be badly arranged for both individual well-being and societal well-being.

Understanding Restrictive Eating Plans
At its center, a restrictive eating plan incorporates through and diminishing caloric affirmations, confining certain food bunches, or taking after strict eating plans. These plans can take distinctive shapes:

1. Caloric Restriction:
Diets that advocate for certainly reducing day-by-day caloric affirmations, frequently to levels underneath what is considered restorative fitting for kept-up prosperity.

2. Irregular Fasting:
Cycling between periods of eating and fasting, with predominant assortments such as the 16/8 procedure (16 hours fasting, 8 hours eating window) or substitute day fasting.

3. Transfer Diets:
Clearing the entirety of food bunches, such as gluten, dairy, or carbohydrates, underneath the conviction that these nourishment are inalienably damaging or cause weight change.

4. Liquid Diets:
Exhausting because it was liquids, such as juices or dinner substitution shakes, for extended periods to realize quick weight mishap.

While shields of these plans regularly tout benefits such as weight mishaps, moved forward metabolic well-being, or progressed mental clarity, the reality is more nuanced. For various individuals, particularly those powerless to cluttered eating behaviors or mental inconvenience, restrictive diets can trigger a cascade of negative outcomes that compromise huge prosperity and well-being.

The Physiological Impact
From a point of view, the human body depends on a balanced affirmation of supplements to function in a perfect world. Essential vitamins, minerals, proteins, fats, and carbohydrates are not fair fuel but basic components that back cellular work, hormone era, and organ prosperity. When subjected to drawn-out caloric restriction or dietary ungainliness, the body begins flexible rebellious to moderate vitality, which can lead to:

Metabolic Quiet:
Lessened imperatives is utilized as the body endeavors to protect imperatives in response to reduced caloric affirmations, making weight mishaps more troublesome.

Supplement Insufficiency:
Inadequately admissions of crucial supplements vital for safe work, bone prosperity, and cognitive execution, growing the chance of need and related prosperity issues.

Muscle Misfortune:
To induce essentials, the body may break down muscle tissue for protein, driving the hardship of slant muscle mass and decreased metabolic rate.

In expansion, restrictive eating plans can exasperate hormonal alter, particularly in women, influencing regenerative well-being and contributing to unusual menstrual cycles or amenorrhoea. These physiological changes not as it were debilitate the anticipated benefits of weight mishaps but pose long-term perils to common well-being.

The Impact of Bad Eating Habits on Health: A Comprehensive Analysis

Eating habits play an important role in determining our overall health and well-being. Poor food choices and eating habits can significantly impact many different aspects of health, leading to short- and long-term consequences. In this comprehensive analysis, we look at different unhealthy eating habits that can harm health, considering their physiological, psychological, and social impacts. By understanding these factors, we aim to highlight the importance of making wise food choices and adopting healthy eating habits.

How we eat directly affects results in our health. In today's rapidly evolving world, the prevalence of unhealthy eating habits is increasing, further contributing to the global burden of chronic diseases such as obesity, diabetes, and cardiovascular disease to name a few. Cancer. Understanding the underlying causes and effects of these unhealthy habits is essential to promoting healthier lifestyles and reducing the incidence of preventable diseases.

Types of Unhealthy eating habits

Consuming too much-processed food

Processed foods are altered from their natural state to ensure safety and convenience. Beneficial or has a shelf life and often contains high levels of sugar, unhealthy fats, and sodium.

1. Health Impact: Regular consumption can lead to weight gain and increase the risk of heart disease, diabetes and other chronic diseases.

2. Skipping meals: intentionally avoiding regular meals, often due to time constraints or misguided weight control efforts.

3. Health effects: Disrupts metabolism, causes nutrient deficiencies and can lead to overeating later in the day.

4. Consuming too much sugar: Consuming large amounts of added sugar found in sugary drinks, desserts, and processed foods.

5. Health Impact: Linked to obesity, type 2 diabetes, dental problems and increased inflammation in the body.

6. Health Impact: This can lead to weight gain, poor body image and a cycle of unhealthy eating behaviors.

7. Mindless eating: Eating without paying attention to portion sizes, hunger cues or the nutritional quality of the food.

8.Health impacts: Often leads to overeating, weight gain and Poor digestion

9. Late-night snacks: Eat snacks or large meals at night, right before bed.

10. Impact on health: Disrupts sleep, affects digestion and can contribute to weight gain.

11. Lack of variety: Limited food choices, leading to nutritional deficiencies and monotonous diets.

12. Health effects: Increased risk of micro-nutrient deficiencies and reduced overall nutrient intake.

Psychological Effects

1. Obesity and weight gain

Related to bad habits: Consuming too much-processed food, consuming too much sugar, and emotional eating contribute to excess calories and weight gain.

2.Health risks: Obesity increases the risk of cardiovascular disease and diabetes. , joint problems and some cancers.

3. Nutritional deficiencies

Related to bad habits: Skipping meals, lack of variety and thoughtless eating can lead to not getting enough essential nutrients like vitamins, minerals and minerals.

4.Health risks: Weakens the immune system, impairs cognitive function and affects overall physical health.

5.Digestive problems

Related to bad habits: Late night snacking, over-consumption of processed foods and lack of fiber contribute to digestive problems such as constipation, bloating and acid reflux.
Health risks: Chronic digestive problems can affect nutrient absorption and quality of life.

5. Mental health
Linked to bad habits: Emotional eating, lack of a balanced diet, a poor eating habits affect mood regulation and mental health.
> Health risks: Increased risk of depression, anxiety and other mental health disorders.

Economic and social consequences

1. Impact on health-care costs

Link to bad habits: The increasing incidence of diet-related chronic diseases increases health-care costs.

2. Well-being care Burden:

Places strain on well-being care frameworks all-inclusive, influencing both open and private divisions.

3. Efficiency and Quality of Life
- Connect to Awful Propensities:
Destitute dietary choices and related well-being issues decrease efficiency and reduce quality of life.

4.Financial Affect:
Misfortune of workdays due to ailment and decreased proficiency influence financial efficiency.

5. Social Standards
Interface to Awful Propensities:
Social impacts and societal standards can propagate undesirable eating propensities.

6.Well-being Value:
Incongruities in getting nutritious nourishment and instruction on solid eating contribute to well-being imbalances.

Methodologies for Receiving Solid Eating Propensities

1. Instruction and Mindfulness
Advancing Dietary Proficiency:
Enabling people to create educated nourishment choices through instruction on sustenance names, feast arranging, and cooking abilities.

2. Behavioral Mediation
Cognitive Behavioral Treatment:
Tending to enthusiastic eating designs and advancing careful eating hones.
Supper Timing and Parcel Control:
Empowering standard dinners, adjusted parcel sizes, and careful eating propensities.

3 . Arrangement and Natural Changes
Nourishment Approach Backing:
Executing controls to diminish sugar substances in handled nourishment and advance more beneficial nourishment situations.

Community Activities:
Supporting neighborhood agribusiness, farmers' markets, and community gardens to extend access to new, nutritious nourishment.

Awful eating propensities have far-reaching suggestions for well-being, influencing people, communities, and social orders at huge. By tending to these propensities through instruction, behavioral interventions, and policy changes, we can advance more advantageous ways of life and mitigate the burden of diet-related illnesses. Engaging people with the information and assets to form positive dietary choices is fundamental for accomplishing superior well-being results and progressing quality of life universally.

CHAPTER 5

THE FOOD GUIDELINES

Food guidelines serve as essential standards for people and communities to create educated choices about their diet. These rules are outlined by well-being organizations and governments around the world to advance well-being, avoid illnesses, and keep up general well-being through ideal nourishment. Understanding and following these rules can altogether affect one's physical and mental well-being, life span, and quality of life.

Significance of Taking after Nourishment Rules

1. Dietary Simpleness:
Nourishment rules guarantee that people get basic supplements fundamental for development, improvement, and support of substantial capacities.

2. Malady Anticipation:
Legitimate nourishment can diminish the hazard of incessant infections such as heart infection, diabetes, and certain cancers.

3.Weight Administration:
Rules advance a adjusted slim down that underpins sound weight support and diminishes the hazard of corpulence.

4. In general Well-being:
A nutritious diet contributes to better vitality levels, temperament steadiness, and cognitive work.

Components of Nourishment Rules
1. Essential Standards

Assortment:
Expend a wide run of nourishment to guarantee admissions of assorted supplements.

- Adjust: Keep up an adjustment between diverse nourishment bunches (e.g., natural products, vegetables, grains, proteins).

- Balance: Hone parcel control and restrain admissions of nourishment tall in fats, sugars, and salt.

- Hydration: Drink an satisfactory sum of water day by day.

2. Nourishment Bunches and Suggested Immaterial

- Natural products and Vegetables: Wealthy in vitamins, minerals, and fiber; suggested everyday servings shift by age and sexual orientation.

- Grains:Emphasize entire grains for fiber and supplements; select entirety wheat, oats, quinoa, etc.

- Proteins:Incorporate incline meats, poultry, angle, beans, nuts, and seeds; shift protein sources for different supplements.

- Dairy:Choose low-fat or fat-free dairy items for calcium and vitamin D; options like invigorated soy drain are appropriate for those who are lactose narrow-minded.

3. Fats and Oils
- Solid Fats:
Select unsaturated fats (e.g., olive oil, avocados, nuts) over immersed and trans fats.
- Parcel Control:Restrain utilization of fats and oils to direct sums to preserve general calorie adjust.
4. Sugar and Salt
- Constrain Included Sugars:Diminish admissions of sugary refreshments, candies, and prepared nourishment tall in included sugars.
- Sodium Decrease:Diminish utilization of high-sodium nourishment (e.g., handled meats and canned soups) to lower the chance of hypertension.

5. Hydration
Water:Drink a satisfactory sum of water day by day; the prescribed admissions shifts based on components like climate and physical action level.

Viable Tips for Actualizing Nourishment Rules
1. Supper Arranging:
Arrange adjusted suppers joining an assortment of nourishment bunches.
2. Perusing Names:
Get nourishment names to create educated choices of approximate bundles of foods.
3. Cooking Strategies:
Utilize solid cooking strategies like steaming, heating, or flame broiling rather than singing.
4. Careful Eating:

Pay consideration to starvation and totality prompts to dodge indulging.

5. Eating Out:

Select more beneficial choices when feasting out by selecting flame broiled things, servings of mixed greens, or vegetable-based dishes.

Social and Person Contemplation

- Social Differences:Adjust nourishment rules to social inclinations and conventions whereas keeping up wholesome simpleness.

- Extraordinary Dietary Needs: Consider person well-being conditions or dietary inclinations (e.g., vegetarianism, gluten intolerance) when applying nourishment rules.

Challenges and Discussions

- Clashing Data:Distinctive sources may offer clashing exhortation on certain nourishment or supplements.

- Availability: Accessibility and reasonableness of nutritious nourishment can be restricted in certain locales or communities.

- Individual Inclinations: Person taste inclinations and propensities may impact adherence to nourishment rules.

Following to nourishment rules is significant for keeping up ideal well-being and well-being. By understanding the standards of adjusted nourishment, making educated nourishment choices, and receiving solid eating propensities, people can essentially progress their quality of life and decrease the hazard of persistent infections. Nonstop upgrades and instruction approximately nourishment rules offer assistance to address rising well-being concerns and guarantee that dietary suggestions reflect the most recent logical proof.

Joining these rules into everyday life requires devotion and exertion but pays off in made strides in well-being results and improved general wellness for people and communities alike.

This directly gives a comprehensive diagram of nourishment rules, covering their significance, components, down-to-earth tips, and considerations. Executing these rules can engage people to create more advantageous nourishment choices and lead an adjusted way of life.

Most of us have probably seen the food guidelines. Growing up, the food setup was often used as a guide to help us know how much and what types of foods we should eat each day to maintain a healthy lifestyle.

Of course, there is still Evidence showing that the food pyramid is very flexible, but in general, if you can look at the food pyramid, you will have a general idea of what is acceptable in a healthy diet. strong and nutritious. Even though it can sometimes be so controversial, there are still basic foods that are still good. Maybe one you create yourself. Many would argue that eating as many grains as the food pyramid suggests is no longer considered the healthiest thing to do.

In fact, with the recent outbreak of celiac disease, Many people promote a grain-free diet and healthy lifestyle as the healthiest choice.
Instead of relying on the food pyramid to determine what is healthy to eat healthy, try looking at

your personal experiences with food and go from there. Some people are healthier when they eat more whole grains, others are not. Use your best judgment here so you can take steps in the right direction for your health.

The standard food pyramid recommends the following:

•Rice, cereals, pasta and bread, can represent up to 11 servings per day.
•For vegetables and fruit, you should eat three to five servings.
•As for their eggs, you can eat about two or three servings a day, as long as you don't have an allergy or lactose intolerance.

When it comes to meat and beans as well as other things like nuts, fish, or poultry, you should consume two or three servings a day.
• Unsurprisingly, sugars, fats and oils come out on top. Because you shouldn't have too many of these. Instead, use them only when necessary to ensure your healthiest possible lifestyle.

Again, this only refers to the standard food guidelines . Depending on your specific needs and dietary functions, you may need to modify this yourself. But if you don't have any specific requirements, here is a benchmark for a food pyramid that can be used to your greatest benefit to create a healthier lifestyle.

CHAPTER 6

Food as Medicine: A Guide to a Healthy Life

In recent years, the concept of food as medicine has received significant attention, highlighting how food choices can affect our health and well-being. This guide explores different foods that not only nourish the body but also provide medicinal benefits that support a healthier lifestyle.

1. Platform: Whole Foods
Whole foods are gradually prepared and left over most of their natural benefits. This category includes fruits, vegetables, whole grains, nuts, seeds, and legumes. They are contain with minerals, antioxidants and vitamins that promote healthy life.

Benefits:
- High Nutrient Density: Whole foods provide essential nutrients without excess calories.
- Rich in fiber: They are rich in fiber, supporting digestive

health and reducing the risk of chronic diseases.
- Antioxidant properties: Many whole foods are rich in antioxidants, which help fight oxidation stress and inflammation.

2. Fruits and Vegetables

Fruits and vegetables are at the heart of a healthy diet. They are rich in vitamins, minerals, and phytonutrients which can help prevent diseases.

Key Players:
- Berries: Blueberries, strawberries, and raspberries are high in antioxidants, particularly flavonoids, which are linked to improved heart health and cognitive function.
- Leafy Greens: Spinach, kale, and Swiss chard are loaded with vitamins A, C, K, and calcium, supporting bone health and reducing the risk of osteoporosis.
- Cruciferous Vegetables: Broccoli, Brussels sprouts, and cauliflower contain sulforaphane, which has been shown to have anti-cancer properties.

3. Whole Grains

Whole grains are great sources of fiber, B vitamins, and complex carbs. Examples of these include quinoa, brown rice, and oats.
- Heart Health: Consuming whole grains can lower cholesterol levels and reduce the risk of heart disease.
- Blood Sugar Control: They help regulate blood sugar levels, making them ideal for managing diabetes.
- Satiety: High in fiber, whole grains promote fullness, aiding in weight management.

4. Healthy Fats

Not all fats are created equal. Healthy fats, such as those found in avocados, nuts, seeds, and olive oil, provide numerous health benefits.

Benefits:
-Anti-Inflammatory: Omega-3 fatty acids from sources like

flax seeds, walnuts, and fatty fish reduce inflammation and support heart health.
- Brain Health: Healthy fats are essential for brain function, improving memory and cognitive performance.
- Skin Health: Fats nourish the skin, keeping it hydrated and reducing signs of aging.

5. Legumes

Chickpeas, lentils, and beans are great plant-based sources of fiber, protein, and other essential elements.

Benefits:
- Heart Health: Regular consumption of legumes is associated with lower cholesterol levels and improved heart health.
- Weight Management: Their high fiber content promotes satiety, helping with weight control.
- Blood Sugar Stability: Legumes help stabilize blood sugar levels, making them beneficial for those with diabetes.

6. Spices and Herbs

Spices and herbs are often overlooked but can have profound health benefits.
Key Spices:
- Turmeric: Known for its anti-inflammatory nature and antioxidant properties, turmeric comprises curcumin. It could enhance joint health and lower the chance of developing chronic illnesses.
- Ginger: Helps with digestive issues and has anti-inflammatory effects. It's also effective in reducing nausea.
- Garlic: Known for its heart-healthy benefits, garlic can lower blood pressure and cholesterol levels.

7. Fermented Foods

Fermented foods, such as yogurt, kimchi, sauerkraut, and kombucha, are rich in probiotics, which support gut health.

Benefits:
- Digestive Health: Probiotics enhance gut microbiota, aiding

digestion and nutrient absorption.
- Immune Support: A healthy gut microbiome is linked to improved immune function.
- Mental Health: Emerging research suggests a connection between gut health and mental well-being, potentially reducing anxiety and depression.

8. The Potency of Seeds and Nuts

Nuts and seeds are high in nutrients and a good source of fiber, protein, and healthy fats.

Advantages:
- Heart Health: Eating nuts regularly lowers cholesterol and lowers the risk of heart disease.
- Weight Control: Nuts' satiating qualities can help with weight management, even though they are high in calories.
- Nutrient Boost: Rich in vitamins E, magnesium, and selenium, nuts and seeds promote several body processes.

9. The Function of Dairy (or Other Options)

For healthy bones, dairy products and their fortified counterparts are great sources of calcium and vitamin D.

Advantages
- Bone Strength: Dairy products high in calcium and vitamin D promote bone density and lower the incidence of fractures.
- Protein Source: Dairy products include high-quality protein, which is necessary for the upkeep and repair of muscles.
Probiotics: Fermented dairy products, such as yogurt, also provide probiotic benefits.

10. Hydrating and herbal teas

Although often overlooked, staying hydrated is essential for overall health. Herbal teas may provide additional benefits.

Benefits:
- Detoxification: herbal teas such as dandelion and ginger support

liver function and detoxification.

- Antioxidant effects: green tea is rich in catechins, whose effects have been linked to reducing cancer risk and improving metabolism.

- Hydration: Staying hydrated is key essential for all body functions, including digestion and temperature regulation.

Food as medicine isn't just about individual foods; it involves a comprehensive approach to diet and lifestyle. Incorporating a variety of nutrient-rich foods, staying hydrated, and practicing mindful eating can provide lasting health benefits.

Incorporating these foods into your daily diet can help you achieve optimal health, prevent chronic disease, and improve your quality of life. Harness the power of food as medicine and nourish your body for a healthier future.

In the same way that not eating healthy can make you sick, eating healthy foods can oftentimes cure you of illness and provide you with relief when you are suffering.

Moreover, it can serve as a prevention against disease. There has been an entire method of healing around India for thousands of years called Aryuveda.

This ancient healing style is utilized to treat any illness simply by changing your diet. Food is the medicine that has helped to keep the people of India alive for centuries.

Furthermore, it is still relevant today. A lot of cures are just good meals that may feed your body from the inside out and have anti-inflammatory qualities. Healthy food choices have been shown to affect everything from cancer to infections.

And it is now more evident than ever with this age-old healing technique.

Naturally, a lot of contemporary technology will disapprove of these techniques as they haven't been well studied by scientists, but a lot of it has been used for thousands of years and will still have an effect on the body.

Whether you subscribe to traditional medical wisdom or not, there's no denying that your diet has a major influence on your susceptibility to disease. Your body will be stronger and more resilient to disease and infection if you consume a healthy diet than if you are starved on a typical American diet.

Without the proper vitamins and minerals in your body, it can be almost impossible to fight off the negative effects of illness. Sometimes, it can even cause illness. If you are eating unhealthy unprocessed foods, certain types of these foods can lead to illnesses and make you more susceptible to certain types of cancer as well. Although cancer is still being researched and has not fully been understood by the scientific community well enough to cure it, there are many instances of people who were able to live long and healthy lives simply by changing the way they need it.

Healthy eating can alleviate the symptoms of many difficult-to-treat diseases, such as multiple sclerosis. the fuel and resources they need to be strong. And they will do it to the best of their ability.

However, your body won't be able to fight back as effectively as it could if you are deliberately undermining it with poor nourishment. You must pay attention to how you are feeding your body because of this. If you don't make proactive and conscious choices about the food you eat, you could be setting yourself up for failure that you may regret.

Chapter 7

The Health Eating Vegetables

Eating vegetables is crucial to a solid diet and has various benefits that contribute to general well-being. Vegetables are rich in vitamins, minerals, and fiber, whereas they are low in calories and fat. Here's a closer see at how consolidating vegetables into your day-by-day suppers can advance a more beneficial way of life.

Supplement Thickness

Vegetables are nutrient-dense, meaning they give a tall sum of supplements relative to their calorie substance. This can be especially useful for keeping up a solid weight and avoiding weight. Key supplements found in vegetables include:

Vitamins:
Numerous vegetables are rich in fundamental vitamins such as A, C, K, and a few B vitamins, which back resistant work, skin well being, and vitality digestion system.
- Minerals:
Vegetables give vital minerals like potassium, magnesium, and calcium, which are crucial for bone well-being, heart work, and muscle withdrawal.
- Cancer prevention agents
Numerous vegetables are tall in antioxidants, which offer assistance to combat oxidation push within the body and decrease the chance of constant illnesses.

Stomach related Well being
The fiber substance in vegetables plays a pivotal part in stomach-related well-being. Dietary fiber makes a difference to:
- Advance Normality:
Fiber includes bulk to stool and encourages normal bowel developments, diminishing the hazard of stoppage.
- Back Intestine Well being:
A fiber-rich diet can cultivate a sound intestine micro-biome, which is connected to progressed assimilation and resistant work.

Weight Administration

Consolidating more vegetables into your count calories can help in weight administration. Their tall fiber and water content help you feel full, which can diminish general calorie admissions. Additionally, low-calorie vegetables can be devoured in bigger amounts, permitting for fulfilling suppers without intemperate calorie utilization.

Heart Well being

Standard vegetable utilization is related to a diminished chance of heart infection. Vegetables can offer assistance to:

- Lower Blood Weight:
Tall potassium levels in vegetables can offer assistance oversee blood weight, contributing to heart well-being.

- Decrease Cholesterol Levels:
Certain vegetables, particularly those high in solvent fiber, can offer assistance in lowering LDL (awful) cholesterol levels.

Illness Avoidance:
Eating a slim down wealthy in vegetables has been connected to a lower chance of a few constant infections:

- Sort 2 Diabetes:
A plant-based eat less can move forward affront affect ability and offer assistance control blood sugar levels.

- Cancer:
A few things propose that a tall admission of vegetables may diminish the chance of certain cancers due to the nearness of phytonutrients and cancer prevention agents.

Skin Wellbeing
The vitamins and cancer prevention agents in vegetables contribute to solid skin. For example:
- Vitamin C:
Imperative for collagen generation and skin repair.

- Beta-Carotene:
Found in orange and yellow vegetables, it can offer assistance secure the skin from sun harm.

Mental Well-Being
There's rising proof that a eat less rich in vegetables can emphatically affect mental well-being. Nutrient-rich nourishment back brain work and may lower the chance of cognitive decrease. A few consider proposing that diets rich in natural products and vegetables are related to lower rates of misery and anxiety.

How to Consolidate More Vegetables
To procure the benefits of vegetables, consider the taking after tips:
1. Include Vegetables in Each Supper:
Incorporate an assortment of vegetables in your breakfast, lunch, and supper.

2. Snack on Vegetables:
Keep crude veggies on hand for good snacks.

3. Attempt Unused Formulas:
Test with diverse cooking strategies, such as broiling, steaming, or flame broiling to improve flavors.

4. Develop Your Possess:
On the off chance that conceivable, developing your possess vegetables can empower utilization and appreciation for new deliver.

Joining an assortment of vegetables into your eat-less advances various well-being benefits, from improved supplement admissions and way better assimilation to decreased malady hazards and moved forward mental well-being. By making vegetables a staple in your dinners, you'll be able to cultivate a more beneficial way of life that supports your well-being both presently and in the future.

This diagram can be extended with particular ponders, nitty gritty supplement profiles, supper plans, or individual anecdotes to reach your particular objective. Let me know in case you wish any particular segments created to assist!

Vegetables are one of the foremost under-sung nourishment in presence, particularly when it comes to the standard American eat less. Most individuals do not realize how important it is to supply the body with the vitamins and minerals that vegetables and vegetables alone can give. Now and then, individuals will see vegetables as a way of progressing their excellence, but when it comes to making strides in their well-being, they become to some degree involved.

Be that as it may, presently simply here and reading this book, it is secure to expect that you simply are willing and able to require into thought why it is critical to eat vegetables. Here are some of the finest reasons to supply yourself with vegetables daily as a portion of your count calories.

To begin with, of all, the body needs fiber to be freed of excess waste. Without a way to discover the squander together and dispense with it, it remains stuck within the body and can contribute to weight pick up and other potential complications.
Fiber is greatly imperative for other reasons as well. It can assist you in anticipating your blood cholesterol from rising and can indeed.

Avoid heart malady, or at least lower the chances of suffering from it.

Folic corrosive is additionally present in vegetables, and after you give your body this substance, it can generate your ruddy blood cells. This could be exceptionally critical in making a difference to avoid iron deficiency from happening and can be exceptionally useful to ladies in particular, who tend to require this substance amid pregnancy and monthly cycle.

Vegetables are also normally high in numerous vitamins, such as A and C, which offer assistance in battling disease and keep the body solid. It can assist you in speeding up the mending handle and assimilating press, which is another way of making a difference to combat and avoid frailty from happening. Vitamins are high in potassium and this can be exceptionally valuable since it prevents the body from surrendering to high blood weight.

Vegetables have been demonstrated to diminish the chance of strokes and other heart-related complications. They can prevent kidney stones from creating and avoid the crumbling of bone matter. Filling yourself up with vegetables is a great way to assist you oversee sort II diabetes and weight.

Not as it were, but it can assist you to remain solid in the battle against cancer and cancer avoidance. Maybe one of the most

Redeeming qualities around eating vegetables is the reality that they are exceptionally moo in fat and are not calorie-dense.

This implies merely eating as many vegetables as you want to without having to worry too much approximately picking up weight. Snacking on vegetables could be an incredible way to help you decrease starvation desires and remain centered on a sound lifestyle.

There are so numerous great things about vegetables. Shockingly, they are so uncommon to come by within the standard American eat less. One of the best ways that you just can help yourself dodge high-fat tall sugar and high-salt handled nourishment is by strolling around the exterior of your basic needs store to begin with.

Go along the fresh produce area so that you just are making cognizant choices in giving your body sound new vegetable alternatives instead of skipping to the conclusion and cheating by buying pasta and other prepared nourishment that are moo in really nutritious vegetable substances.

Sound eating begins with making the choices to feed your body, and there are few things more feeding than vegetables.

Ready to frequently lose our taste for sound nourishment because of undesirable and destitute eating propensities early in life, or even self-imposed afterward in life, but it is simple to urge back on track. Make time in your life for vegetables. They may take a little bit longer to plan, but the benefits are worth it.

Chapter 8

FRUIT-EATING NOURISH OUR BODY

In later a long time, the significance of consolidating natural products into our everyday diets has picked up significant consideration. Natural products are not fair scrumptious; they are pressed with fundamental vitamins, minerals, fiber, and cancer prevention agents that advance general well-being and healthy life. This comprehensive investigation will dig into how natural product utilization can lead to progressed well-being results, counting upgraded safe work, superior assimilation, weight administration, and decreased hazard of constant infections.

Supplement Thickness of Natural products

One of the essential reasons natural products are celebrated in sustenance science is their supplement thickness. Natural products are moo in calories but tall in basic supplements, making them a perfect choice for keeping up an adjusted slim down.

1. Vitamins and Minerals:
Natural products are rich in vitamins such as vitamin C, which bolsters the safe framework and skin well being, and a few B vitamins that help in the vitality digestion system. Minerals like potassium, found in bananas and oranges, play an imperative part in keeping up solid blood weight levels.

2. Cancer prevention agents:
Numerous natural products are high in cancer prevention agents,

which offer assistance in combating oxidation stretch within the body. Berries, for occurrence, are rich in flavonoid that can diminish irritation and lower the chance of unremitting conditions such as heart malady.

3. Dietary Fiber:
Natural products are an amazing source of dietary fiber, which helps in absorption and makes a difference keep up a sound weight. Fiber can lower cholesterol levels and direct blood sugar, which is especially useful for people with diabetes.

Safe Framework Back

A solid resistant framework is pivotal for by and large well being, and natural products play a critical part in upgrading safe work.

1. Vitamin C:
Natural products like oranges, strawberries, and kiwi are inexhaustible in vitamin C, which is known for its immune-boosting properties. This vitamin makes a difference fortify the generation of white blood cells, basic for battling contamination.

2. Antioxidant Properties:
The cancer prevention agents found in natural products offer assistance to decrease aggravation and combat free radicals that can debilitate the safe framework. Customary utilization of antioxidant-rich natural products may lead to a diminished rate of sickness.

3. Hydration:
Numerous natural products, such as watermelon and cucumber, have tall water substances, contributing to hydration. Legitimate hydration is imperative for ideal immune function and by and large well-being.

Stomach related Well being

Keeping up a solid stomach-related framework is fundamental

for supplement assimilation and in general well-being. Natural products contribute essentially to stomach-related well-being in a few ways.

1. Dietary Fiber:
As specified previously, natural products are rich in fiber, which helps assimilation by advancing normal bowel developments and anticipating clogging. Solvent fiber, found in apples and pears, makes a difference control blood sugar levels and bringing down cholesterol.

2. Common Chemicals:
Certain natural products, like pineapples and papayas, contain normal stomach-related chemicals that can offer assistance break down proteins and encourage absorption.

3. Intestine Well being:
A diet rich in natural products bolsters a sound intestine micro-biome, which is pivotal for stomach-related well-being. Fiber acts as a prebiotic, nourishing advantageous intestine microbes that contribute to an adjusted micro-biome.

Weight Administration

In an age where weight rates are on the rise, joining natural products into the count of calories can be an accommodating methodology for weight administration.

1. Low-Calorie Choices:
Natural products are normally moo in calories, permitting people to appreciate bigger parcels without over-the-top calorie intake. This can be useful for those attempting to lose or keep up weight.

2. Satiety:
The tall fiber substance in natural products can advance sentiments of totality, decreasing the probability of indulging. Eating natural products as snacks can fulfill sweet longings without turning to undesirable alternatives.

3. Solid Snacking:
Supplanting prepared snacks with natural products can lead to more beneficial dietary propensities. For occurrence, swapping chips for an apple or a modest bunch of berries can give supplements and fiber while fulfilling starvation.

Unremitting Malady Anticipation

Investigate reliably appears that a eat less diet in natural products is related to a lower hazard of different inveterate infections.

1. Heart Illness:
Customary natural product utilization is connected to diminished blood weight and lower cholesterol levels, both of which are vital in avoiding heart infection. The fiber, potassium, and cancer prevention agents found in natural products contribute to cardiovascular well-being.

2. Diabetes:
Natural products have a moo glycemic file, which implies they have a negligible effect on blood sugar levels when devoured in control. The fiber substance too makes a difference in controlling blood sugar levels, making natural products a shrewd choice for those with diabetes.

3. Cancer:
Various ponders propose that eating less wealthy in natural products may lower the chance of certain sorts of cancer. The cancer prevention agents and phytochemicals found in natural products can secure cells from harm and repress cancer cell development.

4. Stroke:
A slim-down tall in natural products, especially citrus natural products and berries, has been related to a lower chance of stroke. The supplements in these natural products back vascular well-being and decrease irritation.

MENTAL HEALTHY BENEFITS

Natural products are not as it were useful for physical well-being but moreover play a part in mental well-being.

1. Disposition Direction:
Certain natural products, like bananas, contain tryptophan, which can boost serotonin levels and make strides in temperament. A count of calories rich in natural products has been connected to lower levels of sadness and uneasiness.

2. Cognitive Work:
Cancer prevention agents in natural products may secure the brain from oxidation stretch and irritation, possibly diminishing the chance of cognitive decline and demonstrativeness maladies.

3. Vitality Levels:
The characteristic sugars in natural products give a fast source of vitality, making them a fabulous choice for an evening pick-me-up or pre-workout nibble.

Commonsense Tips for Joining Natural products into Your Count calories

1. Assortment is Key:
Point for an assorted extend of natural products to guarantee you get a wide range of supplements. Test with regular natural products and investigate modern assortments.

2. Make Natural products Available:
Keep new natural products unmistakable and effortlessly available in your kitchen or at work to empower sound snacking.

3. Smoothies and Juices:
Mix natural products into smoothies or juices for a fast and nutritious dinner or nibble. In any case, be careful of parcel sizes to dodge intemperate sugar admissions.

4. Fruit-Based Pastries:
Utilize natural products in sweets rather than prepared sugars. Prepared apples, natural product servings of mixed greens, and solidified banana chomps are tasty and advantageous choices.

5. Cook with Natural products:
Consolidate natural products into savory dishes. Include natural products like pineapple, mango, or berries in servings of mixed greens, salsas, or stir-fries for added flavor and nourishment.

The healthy benefits of natural product utilization are tremendous and well-documented. From supporting safe work and stomach-related well-being to advancing weight administration and lessening the chance of inveterate infections, natural products are a crucial component of an adjusted diet. As we endeavor for way better well being and well-being, joining an assortment of natural products into our everyday dinners can lead to significant advancements in our by and large well-being. By grasping the tasty and nutritious nature of natural products, we will develop more advantageous ways of life and improve our quality of life.

Unremitting Malady Anticipation

1. It reliably appears that a reduction in natural product consumption is associated with a lower risk of various chronic diseases. Remember this text:
"It is known that consuming fruits regularly can lead to reduced blood pressure and lower cholesterol levels, both of which are

important in preventing heart disease. The fiber, potassium, and antioxidants found in fruits contribute to cardiovascular health."

2. Diabetes:
"Natural products have a low hypoglycemic index, which means they have a minimal effect on blood sugar levels when consumed in moderation. The fiber content also helps in controlling blood sugar levels, making natural products a smart choice for those with diabetes." Opposes that eating less wealthy natural products may lower the chance of certain sorts of cancer. The cancer prevention agents and phytochemicals found in natural products can secure cells from harm and repress cancer cell development.

3. Stroke:
A study has shown that a diet rich in natural products, especially citrus fruits and berries, is associated with a reduced risk of stroke. The nutrients in these fruits promote vascular health and reduce inflammation.

"Benefits of Mental Well being"

Natural products are not as it were useful for physical well-being but moreover play a part in mental well-being.

1. Disposition Direction:
Certain natural products, like bananas, contain tryptophan, which can boost serotonin levels and make strides in temperament. A count of calories rich in natural products has been connected to lower levels of sadness and uneasiness.

2. Cognitive Work:
Cancer prevention agents in natural products may secure the brain from oxidative stretch and irritation, possibly diminishing the chance of cognitive decline and neurodegenerative maladies.

3. Vitality Levels:
The characteristic sugars in natural products give a fast source of vitality, making them a fabulous choice for an evening pick-me-up or pre-workout nibble.

Remember these tips for incorporating natural products into your diet:

1. Assortment is Key:
Point for an assorted extend of natural products to guarantee you get a wide range of supplements. Test with regular natural products and investigate modern assortments.

2. Make Natural products Available:
Keep new natural products unmistakable and effortlessly available in your kitchen or at work to empower sound snacking.

3. Smoothies and Juices:
Mix natural products into smoothies or juices for a fast and nutritious dinner or nibble. In any case, be careful of parcel sizes to dodge intemperate sugar admissions.

4. Fruit-Based Pastries:
Utilize natural products in sweets rather than prepared sugars. Prepared apples, natural product servings of mixed greens, and solidified banana chomps are tasty and advantageous choices.

5. Cook with Natural products:
Consolidate natural products into savory dishes. Include natural products like pineapple, mango, or berries in servings of mixed greens, salsas, or stir-fries for added flavor and nourishment.

The healthy benefits of natural product utilization are tremendous and well-documented. From supporting safe work and stomach-related well-being to advancing weight administration and lessening the chance of inveterate infections, natural products are a crucial component of an adjusted diet. As we endeavor for way better well being and well-being, joining an assortment of natural products into our everyday dinners can lead to significant advancements in our by and large well-being. By grasping the tasty and nutritious nature of natural products, we will develop more advantageous ways of life and improve our quality of life.

Grapes have been known to be utilized in the combat of cancer as well, especially red-skinned grapes. They are too supportive in battling eye issues and kidney issues. If you endure from disease, berries are particularly supportive. They are tall in cancer prevention agents.

Just make beyond any doubt that you simply are eating natural products and vegetables that are not treated with commercial pesticides, as they can retain these chemicals complicate weight loss, and cause issues within the body.

You'll be able indeed eat dry natural products as a way of substituting unfortunate and sugary snacks and giving your body a sweet nibble that will pack very a dietary punch. Just be conscientious of the sugar levels in dried fruits, since sometimes when they are commercially sold, included sugars make what may well be a sound treat into something that will ultimately assist you in packing on the pounds.

In any case, once you are solidly eating natural products and routinely, natural products can offer assistance to help you with weight misfortune. As long as you're not indulging in things that are high in sugar, the filaments and water substance of natural products will offer assistance to your body feeling full and your cells and organs nourished. The strands and water substance will assist you in dispensing with issues that are contributing to obesity, and by and large, you may feel an immense shift in your vitality levels.

You'll utilize this vitality to exercise and work harder toward a sound way of life. This could be especially effective if you're replacing sugary garbage nourishment with more beneficial natural ones. product choices as you proceed to move on your travel toward superior well-being and well-being.

FRUIT GUIDELINES

fruits are a fundamental portion of an adjusted slim-down, giving crucial supplements, vitamins, and minerals that contribute to general well-being. In any case, with a bunch of alternatives accessible, understanding how to consolidate natural products successfully into our diets can be challenging. This directly investigates the well-being benefits of natural products, suggested servings, choice, capacity, arrangement, and commonsense tips for counting more natural products in day-by-day suppers.

NUTRITIONAL BENEFITS OF FRUITS

1. Vitamins and Minerals:
Natural products are rich in vitamins such as vitamin C, which underpins the safe framework, and vitamin A, pivotal for vision and skin well being. They too give basic minerals like potassium, which makes a difference in direct blood weight.

2. Dietary Fiber:
Numerous natural products are tall in dietary fiber, which helps absorption and can offer assistance keep up a sound weight by advancing a feeling of totality.

3. Cancer prevention agents:
Natural products contain different cancer prevention agents, such as flavonoids and carotenoids, which secure the body from oxidative stretch and may diminish the chance of incessant illnesses like heart illness and cancer.

4. Hydration:
Numerous natural products have tall water substance, contributing to hydration, particularly vital in hot climates or after working out.

Suggested Servings
The USDA's Dietary Rules prescribe that grown-ups devour at the slightest 1.5 to 2 glasses of natural products per day. The precise sum may shift based on age, sex, and level of physical movement.

- 1 glass of fruit can be equivalent to:

- 1 medium apple or banana
- 1 container of berries
- 1 container of chopped natural product
- ½ glass of dried natural product (which is more calorie-dense, so balance is key)

Choosing Natural products

1. Regular and Nearby:
Selecting regular and locally developed natural products can upgrade flavor, diminish natural effects, and frequently lower costs.

2. Natural vs. Ordinary:
Whereas natural natural products are free from engineered pesticides, customary natural products are regularly treated with secure strategies. Washing natural products altogether can moderate pesticide buildups.

3. Entire Natural products vs. Handled:
Entire natural products are by and large more useful than prepared natural product items (like juices and canned natural products in syrup) since they hold their fiber substance and are lower in included sugars.

Capacity of Natural products

1. Refrigeration:
A few fruits, like berries and grapes, advantage from refrigeration, while others, such as bananas and avocados, ought to be put away at room temperature until matured.

2. Maturing:
Certain fruits, including bananas and pears, proceed to mature after being picked. Putting away them in a paper pack can speed up the aging preparation due to the discharge of ethylene gas.

3. Solidifying:
Solidifying natural products can amplify their rack life while

protecting most of their dietary esteem. It's fitting to wash, peel, and cut natural products sometimes recently solidifying for simpler utilization afterward.

Preparation of Fruits

1. Washing:
Continuously wash natural products altogether beneath running water to evacuate soil and buildups. A brush can be utilized for firmer natural products like apples and melons.

2. Peeling and Cutting:
Whereas a few natural products, like apples and pears, are frequently eaten with the skin on (which gives extra fiber), others may require peeling. Guarantee to utilize clean utensils to avoid cross-contamination.

3. Cooking:
A few natural products can be cooked (like apples and peaches), which can modify their surface and flavor, even though cooking may decrease a few vitamins. Utilizing negligible water and cooking briefly can offer assistance preserve nutrients.

Practical Tips for More Fruits

1.Breakfast Boost:
Include cut natural products to cereal, yogurt, or smoothies for included sweetness and nourishment.

2.Snacking:
Keep entire natural products helpful for snacks. They're convenient, making them simple to require on the go.

3.Servings of mixed greens:
Consolidate natural products into servings of mixed greens, such as including strawberries or orange fragments to verdant greens.

4.Pastries: or natural product compotes can serve as solid choices
Utilize natural products as a common sweetener in sweets. Heated

natural products or natural product compotes can serve as sound choices

65

Chapter 9

HEALTH BENEFITS
OF MEAT

Meat is by and large considered one of the essential staple nourishment in an e-mail, but it may be astounding to discover that there are a few meats that are more advantageous than others. Of course, we know the distinction between ruddy meats and white meats. Ruddy meats are more regularly connected to well-being issues and coronary issues, whereas white meats are considered leaner and more beneficial in general.

What a few individuals may be astounded to discover is that other issues make meats unfortunate. Issues such as the things that they are nourished while the creatures are still lively and anti-microbial and hormones which will be infused into them to create them develop quicker or create more drain, at slightest within the case of dairy animals.

These sorts of hormones eventually enter the meat that we devour and can cause issues in our bodies. If we are not honest about the choices that we make when we are choosing our nourishment, they can eventually contribute to destitute well-being in the future, including but not restricted to cancers and hormone changes that can be very weakening.

In any case, on the off chance that you're sure that you're getting your meat from sources that are healthy and don't nourish creatures over steroids and anti-microbial, at that point, you're as of now ahead of the diversion. In case not, try to do a little research about neighborhood places where you'll get meat that's untainted by a few unsafe industry measures.

That being said, indeed considering the healthy meat choices, certain meats are more advantageous than others. One of the most advantageous meats merely can eat, particularly in case you're trying to lose weight, is the angle. Angle is lean and stuffed with supplements. In any case, you have got to be cautious about the source of your angle.

A few angles are raised in undesirable conditions, whereas another angle may come from areas that may be contaminated with mercury. Usually why it is scowled upon for pregnant women to eat fish or shellfish.

But in case you discover a sound source of angle, this will be exceptionally useful for your body. Angle is tall in omega-3 greasy acids, which offer assistance in brain work and memory. Generally, Omega threes are profoundly pined for and the body needs them to operate at its most noteworthy conceivable potential, especially when it comes to mental things.

Chicken that has been raised in a great environment is another incredible choice. Chicken is tall in protein. In reality, it is the most noteworthy in protein of any other meat. They are usually raised in good conditions, or at the slightest bolstered nourishments that will not cause the human body issues the same way a parcel of meat can.

In any case, if you're eating grass hamburgers from a reliable supplier, can moreover be an incredible alternative as well. If you're attending to eat natural chicken, there is by and large less probability of these animals being raised with unsafe carcinogens.

Chickens that have been customarily grown are more often than not nourished nourishments that increment the rate at which they develop, which can lead to genuine well-being issues for the chickens themselves and for the humans that expend them. They are moreover given a huge supply of antidepressants and painkillers, in some cases, indeed arsenic and caffeine.

It is unsafe to expend a parcel of customarily developed meat, but if you'll be able to discover a great provider, at that point you certainly ought to do so.

Turkey is another extraordinary meat since it is tall in selenium. This is something incredible for the body, particularly since it can offer assistance in dispensing with free radicals and other toxic substances.

Again though, you need to undertake to create beyond any doubt that you simply are accepting your meat from reliable sources, since it is standard for ordinarily developed chicken and turkey to be treated additionally and encouraged with unsafe chemicals that unnaturally increment their rate of development and eventually sully human bodies with those chemicals.

Eating meat generally can be exceptionally advantageous for the body, as long as you're not eating meat that comes from perilous and customarily developed strategies. The chemicals that these creatures are frequently subject to our especially dangerous, both to the creatures themselves and to the people who devour them. If you need to eat sound and lose weight, it is way better to maintain a strategic distance from any chemicals that will conclusion up remaining stuck in your body and prevent weight misfortune from happening.

Indeed in case you're not trusting to lose weight, eating sound incorporates dodging anything that may well be perilous to the body, such as the hormones and chemicals that are troublesome to our touchy frameworks. Luckily, there are many sources for healthy meats, whether you need to enjoy chicken, hamburger, or indeed sheep. There are ways that you simply can get solid, ethically raised me to fulfill any longings you may have.

Beyond any doubt! Here's a brief outline of the well being benefits of meat, covering basic supplements, different sorts of meat, and potential well being impacts

Well being Benefits of Meat

Meat may be a noteworthy portion of numerous diets around the world and offers an extent of well-being benefits when expended in balance and as a portion of an adjusted count of calories. Here are a few key focuses enumerating the well being benefits of diverse sorts of meat:

1. Dietary Esteem

Protein Source:

Meat is an amazing source of high-quality protein, which is fundamental for muscle development, repair, and generally substantial work. Proteins are made up of amino acids, a few of which are fundamental and must be obtained through counting calories.

Vitamins:

- B Vitamins:
Meat is rich in a few B vitamins, counting B12, which is vital for nerve work and the generation of DNA and ruddy blood cells.

- Iron:
Ruddy meat, in particular, could be an awesome source of heme press, which is more effortlessly ingested by the body compared to non-heme press from plant sources. Press is imperative for oxygen transport within the blood.

Minerals:

Meat gives critical minerals such as zinc and selenium, both of which play basic roles in immune work, wound recuperation, and cellular digestion system.

2. Sorts of Meat and Their Benefits

Ruddy Meat:

Incorporates meat, sheep, and pork. Ruddy meat is rich in protein, press, and zinc. It moreover contains creatine, which can offer assistance move forward with workout execution.

Poultry:

Chicken and turkey are leaner than ruddy meat, giving protein with a lower fat substance. They are moreover a great source of niacin (B3) and phosphorus.

Angle:

Greasy angles like salmon, mackerel, and sardines are tall in omega-3 greasy acids, which have anti-inflammatory properties and are advantageous for heart well being. Angle moreover contains vitamin D and selenium.

3. Muscle and Bone Well being

Protein admissions from meat bolsters muscle mass, particularly critical as we age. Adequate protein is fundamental for keeping up quality and anticipating sarcopenia (age-related muscle misfortune). Moreover, the phosphorus and vitamin D in meat contribute to bone well being.

4. Cognitive Work

Certain supplements found in meat, especially omega-3 greasy acids from an angle and B vitamins from different meats, are connected to improved cognitive function. These supplements play a part in brain well-being and may offer assistance decrease the hazard of cognitive decrease and neurodegenerative infections.

5. Satiety and Weight Administration

Protein-rich nourishment like meat can upgrade sentiments of totality and diminish by and large calorie admissions. Counting incline meats in suppers can offer assistance with weight administration by advancing satiety and decreasing longings.

6. Metabolic Well being

Normal utilization of incline meat can be the portion of an

adjusted count of calories that underpins metabolic well-being.

 The amino acids found in meat are vital for metabolic forms, counting muscle protein amalgamation, which can improve the general metabolic rate.

7. Contemplation
Whereas meat has numerous well-being benefits, it's vital to devour it in control and select incline cuts to play down soaked fat admissions. Prepared meats ought to be constrained due to their affiliation with well-being dangers such as cardiovascular illness and certain cancers.
Meat can be a nutritious expansion to an adjusted count of calories, giving fundamental proteins, vitamins, and minerals that bolster general well-being. Choosing incline cuts and adjusting meat utilization with plenty of natural products, vegetables, and entire grains is key to maximizing well-being benefits while minimizing potential dangers.

Chapter 10

THE DEMERIT OF FOOD PROCESSING

It does not come as an astonishment to anyone that prepared nourishments are perilous. What does come as a astonish be that as it may is that they are still permitted out on the racks, despite the devastation that they wreak on our bodies and minds. Eating undesirable nourishment isn't fair a individual choice for a few individuals.

Some of the time, because of the way the economy works, individuals in destitution are constrained to turn to prepared nourishment since they are a cheap and simple way to nourish huge families on a small budget.

The difficult thing around that is that these nourishments eventually cause restorative issues down the line that have taken a toll indeed more cash than it would take to nourish a huge family sound, feasible choices. Eventually, it appears that individuals with small cash are enduring either way.

Indeed if you do not need to nourish a family on a budget, prepared nourishments are essentially unfortunate. A portion of what makes them so addicting is their tall fat and sugar substance.

They are frequently boxed suppers that incorporate pastas and an uncommon sum of sugar. Intemperate sugar is perilous in common, but particularly to individuals who are inclined to creating sort II diabetes. In case you devour sugar and tall sums, you're eventually reaching to over-burden your body and not as it were will you gotten to be corpulent, more than likely, but you also create well being issues.

Sugar can offer assistance speed along the method of diabetes since of the reality that it causes affront resistance to happen which eventually makes it troublesome, in case not outlandish, to control your blood sugar levels.

In case you eat foods like this too much, such as for each dinner, or at least each day, there's bound to be a negative result. Expanding that tall sum of fat and sugar on a steady premise can lead to not as it were diabetes and weight, which are commonly known, but too heart infection and indeed cancer. This is often uncommonly unsafe, and in case conceivable, handled nourishments ought to be maintained a strategic distance from at all costs.

Another peril of eating handled nourishments is that not as it were are they addicting, but they are exceedingly manufactured. Most of the fixings in those nourishments are not feeding the body. Or maybe, they are driving us to feel full while denying our bodies the basic supplements that are required in sound working.

When we are eating a slim down that's bland and not feeding, we are eventually permitting ourselves to be dumbed down. We are not considering appropriately, we are not moving legitimately, and we are not working at her most elevated conceivable potential. All of these things are profoundly harmful and can lead to destitute coordination and indeed misery.

On a few levels, we all know that handled nourishments are not as sound as the sorts of nourishments we ought to be expending on a standard basis. Our bodies know it, indeed if our minds are not mindful. And we endure for it. We have stretched around it.

When we enjoy undesirable nourishments, whether we are dependent on them or not, our bodies know it. And, whether it's a subliminal event or not, we regularly rebuff ourselves. We know that we are doing something off-base. We feel disturbed approximately it and disappointed, indeed on the off chance that we are processing it within the minute.

Handled nourishments are moreover tall in fake colorings that have been demonstrated to be exceedingly carcinogenic. When we are eating nourishments that have settled coloring in it, we are basically gulping color. Would you need to eat hair dye? Not really. But these types

of chemicals are what are utilized in your nourishment. They remain in your body and don't come out. They color your organs on the interior. They are exceedingly unsafe and can lead to cancer.

There moreover full of additives. Handled nourishment remains on the shelf for a long time. Longer than is sound and ordinary. Any

a normal bottle of drain would not final for months on conclusion at a time. It would turn sour and ruin. The same as with cheeses, and the same as with other nourishments that you just discover on the shelves that have long rack lives.

Rack lives are vital for companies to set up since they can create more cash in case their nourishment can remain on the rack longer. They will do anything it takes, whether it is more beneficial not to the human body, to guarantee that they are making the foremost cash conceivable.

Additives frequently incorporate unfortunate and unnatural chemicals and over-the-top sums of salt. Not one or the other which are great for the body at all. Handled nourishment can lead to issues with the heart, and hypertension, because of the intemperate sum of salt shown in these nourishment. Tall blood weight may be a common event among individuals who survive off of prepared nourishment, and corpulence and heart assaults are a few of the number one killers in North America.

This has absolutely everything to do with the standard American eat less. The pitiful portion around it is that indeed on the off chance that you know it is undesirable, the chemicals and tall sugar and fat substance make these handled nourishment greatly addicting.

The body starts to crave them, and it can be almost as perilous as sedate enslavement. Once you are addicted to a nourishment

that's not one or the other feeding nor sound, it can have long-term results on your well-being and improvement.

Another way that prepared nourishment contribute to weight is that we process them distant as well quickly compared to nourishment that are rich in solid dietary fiber. In case we are processing these nourishment rapidly and they are not filling us up since we are not accepting the fiber that gives us the complete feeling, we are not indeed burning the same sum of vitality as we would process sound nourishment.

This implies that we eat more and process less, leading to fast and rapid weight pick-up. The calories shown in your body are much higher once you are on a slim down of handled nourishment. You burn distant more calories after you are eating sound, entire nourishment that are wealthy in dietary filaments.

Shockingly, this implies that individuals who live and subsist on a eat less of handled nourishment are eventually progressing to gain weight whether they need to or not. And they will not give you the same sum of energy because they are not feeding. They are likely to make you tired and drowsy and feel distant as well full since you eat a part more of these undesirable, sugar-filled nourishment without feeling substance or satisfaction.

Handled nourishment isn't metabolized appropriately in our bodies. They are rapidly turned to fat. Not as it were that, but they are tall in fat. They are regularly full of covered-up fat and sugars. Vegetable oil is one of the primary fixings in numerous of these handled suppers,

besides things such as tall fructose corn syrup, which could be a gigantic offender in weight pick up.

On the off chance that each prepared nourishment on the racks contained tall fructose corn syrup, and most of them do, it is no wonder that North America is confronting the most noticeably awful weight scourge in world history. Hydrogenated oils are highly unhealthy since they don't break down.

They stay in your body and get to be consolidated with the fat cells. These oils make fat more difficult to burn off. They are harder to induce freed of, which sort of adamant fat can lead to corpulence exceptionally rapidly. The ingredients in handled nourishment need most of the wholesome esteem that people require in arrange to operate at their highest potential. We require the strands and the vitamins and minerals that are shown in genuine nourishment some time recently ready to genuinely flourish.

On the off chance that you discover that handled nourishment can't be completely dodged, they ought to at slightest be eaten in balance. They are perilous. They can make us feel drowsy, crabby, and despondent in general.

Our minds can go from positive to negative when we go from a sound count of calories and eventually discover ourselves devoured with nothing but handled nourishment that are as well sugary, as well greasy, and unfortunate.

Our bodies need nourishment. The most straightforward and most advantageous thing you'll be able do for yourself is to supply your body with that nourishment. It can be difficult to induce utilized to changing of schedules such as subsisting off of handled nourishment, and it can be very baffling at times.

You've got to spend a parcel more time in the kitchen cooking and taking your well-being and your dinners into thought. But ultimately, eating prepared nourishment is something that can murder you and cut you off from yourself. You're consuming poisons and dodging the nourishment that can act as cancer prevention agents that will give you a chance to induce freed of the squander merely are putting into your body.

Processed foods are the same as junk foods. They are no distinctive. They are more beneficial appearing garbage nourishment. They are snacks in masks. In arrange to end up solid and to feel solid, dodging handled nourishment at all costs is the primary and most successful step that you simply can take. Do not let yourself be tricked by bundling that claims these nourishment are sound.

They are soaked and fat and sugar and salt, and missing in anything that gives your body nourishment. Do everything you'll be able to change your propensity of relying on handled nourishment. Eating sound is easy and conceivable in case you set your intellect to it.

Fair keep in mind the methodology of walking around the basic need store to choose up the new create and meat as opposed to strolling through the paths that are full of perilous and appealing bundling that's stowing away the threats of the processed nourishment inside.

FOOD PROCESSING

Food processing is a multifaceted industry and an essential part of the modern food system. It involves a variety of techniques that transform agricultural raw materials into products suitable for human consumption. This transformation increases food safety, extends shelf life, improves taste and increases usability. However, the process also raises concerns about nutritional quality, additives and environmental impact.

The primary objective of food processing is to ensure food safety by minimizing microbial contamination and preserving the nutritional content of the raw materials. This is achieved through a variety of methods including cleaning, sorting and pasteurization. Cleaning involves removing dirt, debris, and other contaminants from raw materials before processing begins to ensure they meet hygiene standards. Sorting involves separating raw materials based on size, shape, or quality to ensure uniformity and consistency in the final product.

Pasteurization is a common method of killing harmful bacteria and extending the shelf life of products such as milk and fruit juices. The liquid is heated to a specific temperature for a set time and then rapidly cooled to prevent further bacterial growth. This process ensures that the nutritional value of the food is maintained and that it is safe to consume.

Another important aspect of food processing is preservation, which prevents spoilage and extends shelf life. Preservation techniques include canning, freezing, drying, and packaging. Canning involves heating foods in an airtight container to destroy the bacteria and enzymes that cause spoilage. This method is often used for fruits, vegetables, and prepared foods. Freezing slows microbial growth and enzymatic activity, preserving the quality of fresh foods such as meat, seafood, and vegetables.

Drying removes moisture from foods, inhibiting microbial growth and extending their shelf life. They are used for dried fruits, herbs, and spices. Packaging is important in preserving food by protecting it from physical, chemical, and biological damage. It also lists product information such as ingredients, nutritional content, and expiration date.

Food processing also improves food safety through techniques such as fermentation and irradiation.Fermentation uses microorganisms such as bacteria or yeast to convert sugars into acids, alcohol, and gases. This process not only preserves food but also improves its taste, texture, and nutritional value. Examples include yogurt, cheese, and fermented vegetables such as sauerkraut and kimchi.

Irradiation is a food safety technique that uses ionizing radiation to kill bacteria, parasites, and insects. It can also delay the ripening and germination of fruits and vegetables, extending their shelf life. Although radiation is controversial, it is approved in some countries and is considered safe when used within legal limits.

Despite all its benefits, food processing can also affect nutritional quality. Processing methods such as milling and refining can result in the loss of fiber and nutrients from grains, resulting in a less nutritious product. For example, refined flour lacks the fiber and important nutrients found in whole grains. Similarly, excessive heating during processing can destroy heat-sensitive vitamins and enzymes in fruits and vegetables.

In addition, some processing techniques add preservatives, flavor enhancers, and other additives to improve taste, texture, and shelf life. Although these additives are generally considered safe by regulatory authorities, their long-term health effects remain controversial and of concern.

Food processing also has environmental impacts, including energy consumption, waste generation, and water consumption. Energy-intensive processes such as preserving and freezing require large amounts of electricity and fossil fuels, contributing to greenhouse gas emissions and climate change. Waste products generated during processing, such as shells, pods, and trimmings, can strain landfill capacity and cause environmental pollution if not properly disposed of.

To address these concerns, the food processing industry is increasingly focusing on sustainable practices, such as energy-efficient technologies, waste reduction, and recycling. For example, some companies are using renewable energy sources such as solar and wind energy to reduce their carbon footprint. Others are introducing innovative packaging solutions that minimize waste and improve recyclability.

Furthermore, consumer demand for minimally processed and organic foods has led to the development of new processing techniques that maintain nutritional quality while minimizing additives and environmental impact. These include techniques such as high-pressure processing, which uses pressure to preserve food without the application of heat, thereby retaining more nutrients and flavor.

In summary, food processing plays a vital role in the modern food system by ensuring food safety, extending shelf life, and improving convenience. However, there are also concerns about nutritional quality, additives, and environmental impact. By adopting sustainable practices and innovative technologies, the food industry can continue to meet the growing demand for safe, nutritious, and environmentally friendly food.

Chapter 11

Meal Planning

Supper arranging can be one of the single most imperative perspectives for creating a solid way of life. When we are incapable of imagining the long haul of our eating, it can be exceptionally simple to surrender to the enticements of unhealthy nourishments that we have ended up dependent on. Particularly if it is our propensity to eat them instead of eating the nourishments that will feed us.

Feast arranging is a very endeavor. It can be to some degree threatening, particularly to somebody who suffers from organization. If you discover yourself having a difficult time with dinner arranging, do not fuss. There are many ways that you simply can begin to delve into feast arranging that are fun and simple, whether you battle with inventiveness within the kitchen or not.

There are many supper arranging units that you simply can purchase. Numerous of them have the alternative of requesting boxes full of new nourishments to cook with and incorporate formulas merely can utilize. This may be exceptionally supportive in case you're not utilized to cooking, which is regularly the case.

Particularly when destitute eating propensities and an active work plan make it appear troublesome to carve out the time vital in arranging to form full, feeding suppers. The primary step in meal planning is research. If you're going to get yourself sound, you have got to see your alternatives.

Inquiring about formulas is leading, to begin with, put to begin. Amassing a cover full of solid nourishments simply to attempt out can be both fun and instructive. It'll open your mind to several food possibilities you'll have something else jeered at as too troublesome for you to get ready, or possibly educate you on things you had never known some time recently.

Recipes can be exceptionally mind-opening. Particularly when you're curious about making unused discoveries. Cooking can be a hard propensity to induce into, but once you start to master it, you may be shocked by just how much freedom you can discover in putting a feast together for yourself that's both health-conscious and scrumptious!

See formula books and magazines and get an amassing of formulas that merely need to be attempted. Begin with the things that seem the foremost tasty and feeding, and in case you're an amateur within the kitchen, you'll too need to see at the things that appear the most straightforward.

Next, you ought to keep your formulas organized in a simple way that is easy to explore. If you find yourself overpowered by a need for organization, it'll make supper arranging that much more difficult.

Once you are starting a new habit, you need to make beyond any doubt that you simply are doing everything as essentially as conceivable. As well many alterations at once can be requested on your framework, and you ought to continuously attempt to execute small, easy changes until they have become an unused habit.

Make doubt that they are easily available so that when you want to start planning your dinner you'll do so effectively. In case you are employing a cover, you may need to consider laminating the pages or utilizing plastic sleeves, so that if you're utilizing it in the kitchen, they are not influenced by water or other food contamination.

After you organize your formulas, it will offer assistance to put them in a range of breakfast dinners, lunch dinners, supper meals, and snacks. This will assist you in referencing the correct formulas more effortlessly once you start to cook. In case you like, you may indeed organize your binder by day of the week, and have your suppers arranged out for every day and printed out within the folio that way.

There are numerous ways you'll organize your formulas. Do what appears to create the foremost sense to you naturally. Do not constrain yourself to adhere to a sort of organization that doesn't work.

For you. Instep, make beyond any doubt that you simply are doing what works best for you in your own life.

Make beyond any doubt that you simply are taking the time to routinely look for out modern formulas that stand out to you to keep your inventive juices streaming and your kitchen energizing. There are numerous sorts of formulas you'll be able to attempt, and the more you endeavor, the more curiously going on a travel of solid eating can be!

Following, you ought to investigate programs such as Exceed Expectations on Microsoft Office that will assist you in organizing your meal planning. On Exceed Expectations you may discover a plethora of layouts you'll select from to offer assistance yourself arranging your meals by day, time, and week. This could be a tremendously important asset!

If you'd lean toward not exceeding expectations, there are also apps you'll download on your phone tablet, or another gadget to assist you in utilizing your time and assets way better.

You'll indeed go the ancient designed course and purchase a scratch pad that's extraordinarily outlined toward arranging suppers. Typically a vital step in making beyond any doubt your suppers are organized and effectively accessible.

Having a meal plan is greatly accommodating when it comes to embarking upon a journey of healthy eating. Making great propensities takes time and persistence, and it is inescapable simply will slip someplace along the way.

But that doesn't cruel simply need to remain stuck on the ground! It implies that simply aiming to get back up and keep attempting, since giving up is distant less demanding than staying to your plans.

One thing that can truly offer assistance when it comes to supper arranging is staying with the theme. For illustration, a lot of individuals have specific themes like Taco Tuesday or another day that is allowed for a particular type of supper. On the off chance that you think that would assist you in staying on track, feel free to mimic that type of dinner planning. It is done for a reason since it works and it helps to keep things straightforward and streamlined.

It can be very annoying to discover yourself stuck doing a lot of arranging and planning every single week or month, so on the off chance that you want to keep things simple, that can be a great way to do it. You'll have a subject for every other week's dinners, such as taco Tuesday one night and maybe rice and vegetables Tuesday the following, and interchange between them. There's no wrong way to plan your suppers. What you have to make sure you do is to observe and take after through.

Without follow-through, everything else gets to be repetitive and troublesome. Something that can genuinely assist you to succeed at feast arranging is responsibility. On the off chance that you let somebody who knows you and cares about you know that you simply are endeavoring to arrange

Your suppers, ask them in case they would be willing to help you stay in your routine.

They can assist you by inquiring questions approximately how things are going and whether or not you're remaining on track. They may too select to energize you and cheer you on through your endeavors.

Be that as it may, they select to bolster you, and they can be exceptionally fulfilling for both of you. On the off chance that they are a positive and strong person, it can be extraordinary to know that you just have people rallied in your corner who need you to succeed. Fair make beyond any doubt simply are weeding out harmful individuals who bring you down by turning the consideration onto themselves or by making you're feeling as in case it'll be troublesome for you to achieve your objectives.

Beyond any doubt, useful input can be unimaginably valuable, but if you're not looking for helpful criticism, it can at times be poisonous.
Make beyond any doubt you get the contrast between a harmful individual disguised as a steady individual and a steady individual who genuinely needs to see you flourish.

Another way to require responsibility is by taking individual responsibility. Individual responsibility can be accomplished through journaling and self confirmations. Talking to yourself approximately your objectives, what do you do it inside or out boisterous, can be a great way

to help you to remain centered and inquire yourself whether or not you're doing the things that you just hope to achieve.

In the event that you discover that you simply are not, rather than beating yourself up about it, consider your deterrents and move on as you start to reveal them. The only way you may ever be a failure is on the off chance that you are doing not try. In the event that you attempt, everything will ultimately fall into put since you're making an exertion and making positive changes in your life.

Journaling is valuable for many reasons. They can assist you to compose down what you have got eaten and when and how much. This will give you a good idea of what you'll be able practically anticipate from yourself. The things simply are despondent with, you ought to address and take note of. But rather than being irate at yourself for not being a stream right absent, keep in mind that it may be a prepare and you wish to go gradually.

Rather than actualizing a complete alter in schedule and arranging out each feast for the next month once you have never done it before, instead, begin moderate by facilitating into one or two meals a week, and after that gradually adding in the rest as you feel comfortable with the prepare.
Make it something that does not stun your framework. Progressive alter is the foremost lasting. And journaling about your experiences will assist you to reveal your innermost thoughts about the method and things that you simply might not indeed realize were holding you back.

You'll start to sense patterns in your behavior and possibly predict after you discover yourself tempted to get off track and why. On the off chance that you'll distinguish these trigger focuses it will be easier to dodge them in the long run.

Dinner arranging can be a really fun and energizing endeavor. Indeed on the off chance that you aren't the sort who appreciates that sort of organization, it can be exceptionally fulfilling to think almost precisely what you are getting to be putting in your body and take the steps vital to do so. Everyone merits a chance to end up with the most beneficial and most solid adaptation of themselves conceivable, and with supper arranging and a sound dosage of self-esteem, you will be well on your way to a way of life of solid eating.

They can assist you by inquiring questions approximately how things are going and whether or not you're remaining on track. They may too select to energize you and cheer you on through your endeavors.

Be that as it may, they select to bolster you, and they can be exceptionally fulfilling for both of you. On the off chance that they are a positive and strong person, it can be extraordinary to know that you just have people rallied in your corner who need you to succeed. Fair make beyond any doubt simply are weeding out harmful individuals who bring you down by turning the consideration onto themselves or by making you're feeling as in case it'll be troublesome for you to achieve your objectives.

Beyond any doubt, useful input can be unimaginably valuable, but if you're not looking for helpful criticism, it can at times be poisonous.
Make beyond any doubt you get the contrast between a harmful individual disguised as a steady individual and a steady individual who genuinely needs to see you flourish.

Another way to require responsibility is by taking individual responsibility. Individual responsibility can be accomplished through journaling and self confirmations. Talking to yourself approximately your objectives, what you do it inside or out boisterous, can be a great way

to help you to remain centered and inquire yourself whether or not you're doing the things that you just hope to achieve.

In the event that you discover that you simply are not, rather than beating yourself up about it, consider your deterrents and move on as you start to reveal them. The only way you may ever be a failure is on the off chance that you are doing not try. In the event that you attempt, everything will ultimately fall into put since you're making an exertion and making positive changes in your life.

Journaling is valuable for many reasons. They can assist you to compose down what you have got eaten and when and how much. This will give you a good idea of what you'll be able practically anticipate from yourself. The things simply are despondent with, you ought to address and take note of. But rather than being irate at yourself for not being a stream right absent, keep in mind that it may be a prepare and you wish to go gradually.

Rather than actualizing a complete alter in schedule and arranging out each feast for the next month once you have never done it before, instead, begin moderate by facilitating into one or two meals a week, and after that gradually adding in the rest as you feel comfortable with the prepare.
Make it something that does not stun your framework. Progressive alter is the foremost lasting. And journaling about your experiences will assist you to reveal your innermost thoughts about the method and things that you simply might not indeed realize were holding you back.

You'll start to sense patterns in your behavior and possibly predict after you discover yourself tempted to get off track and why. On the off chance that you'll distinguish these trigger focuses it will be easier to dodge them in the long run.

Dinner arranging can be a really fun and energizing endeavor. Indeed on the off chance that you aren't the sort who appreciates that sort of organization, it can be exceptionally fulfilling to think almost precisely what you are getting to be putting in your body and take the steps vital to do so. Everyone merits a chance to end up with the most beneficial and most solid adaptation of themselves conceivable, and with supper arranging and a sound dosage of self-esteem, you will be well on your way to a way of life of solid eating.

Meal Planning

It's a strategic approach to taking control of your diet, saving time, and reducing stress. Whether you want to eat healthier, save money, or simply streamline your daily life, mastering the art of meal planning will change the way you think about food. Here's everything you need to know to become a meal-planning master.

Why Meal Planning is Important

Meal planning isn't just for super-planned people. It's a powerful tool that can benefit everyone, regardless of lifestyle or food preferences. That's why it's important:

1. Eat Healthier: When you plan your meals, you're more likely to make nutritious choices. This helps you avoid unhealthy last-minute options like fast food and heavily processed meals.

2. Save Time: Planning your meals can save you time throughout the week. No more staring at the fridge wondering what to make for dinner or rushing to the store for ingredients you forgot.

3. Reduce Stress: Avoid mealtime stress by knowing in advance what you're going to eat. No more decision fatigue after a long day or frantic searching for a meal.

4. Budget-Friendly: Meal planning helps you stick to your grocery budget by reducing impulse buys and food waste.

5. Variety and Creativity: Contrary to popular belief, meal planning doesn't mean eating the same thing every day. She recommends trying new recipes, flavors, and dishes while still maintaining a balanced diet.

How to Start Meal Planning Like a Pro

Ready to get started on meal planning? To get started, follow these steps:

**1. Decide your destination. **Be clear about your reason for creating a meal plan. Is it for health reasons, to save time, or to stay on a budget? Understanding your goal will determine your approach.

2. Choose your planning method: There are multiple ways to plan your meals, from simple pen and paper to digital apps.

3. Create a Weekly Plan: Start planning your meals for the next week. Consider your schedule. Busy days may call for quick and easy meals, but weekends allow you more time to cook.

4. Collect Recipes: Collect recipes that suit your goals and preferences. Consider factors like prep time, available ingredients, dietary restrictions, etc.

5. Make a Shopping List: Once you have decided on your meal plan, make a shopping list based on the ingredients you will need. Stick to a list to avoid impulse buying.

**6. Prepare Ahead: ** Preparing ingredients ahead of time can save you time during the week. Chop veggies, marinate meat, cook grains, and store them for easy prep later.

7. Stay flexible: Life goes on and plans can change. Have backup options like easy recipes and frozen meals on hand for busy days or unexpected events.

Tips and Tricks for Successful Meal Planning

Here are some additional tips to make meal planning even more effective and fun:

1. Buy in Bulk: Cook large quantities of staples like grains, proteins, and sauces to use for multiple meals throughout the week.

2. Theme Nights: Assign themes to certain days of the week (e.g. Meatless Monday, Taco Tuesday) to simplify and add variety to your meal planning.

3. Make use of leftovers: Plan for leftovers to reduce waste and save time.

4. Involve your family: Get input from your family when planning meals. This ensures that everyone's preferences are taken into account and creates a sense of unity.

5. Keep it simple: Not every meal needs to be elaborate. Quick and easy recipes can be delicious and nutritious too.

6. Use seasonal ingredients: Incorporating seasonal ingredients into your meal plan will result in fresher, tastier meals and potentially cost savings.

7. Review and Adjust: Regularly review your meal planning process to see what's working and what you can improve. Adjust your approach if necessary.

Overcoming Common Challenges

Though meal planning has many benefits, it's not without its challenges. To overcome common obstacles:

1. Lack of Time: Start small and gradually build up your meal-planning skills. Planning just a few meals a week can make a big difference.

2. Recipe Fatigue: Vary your recipes regularly and try new dishes to keep them interesting.

3. Impulse Eating: Keep healthy snacks on hand to curb cravings and resist the temptation to make impulsive food decisions.

4. Dietary Restrictions: With careful planning and creativity, you can accommodate a variety of dietary needs and preferences when planning your meals.

5. Acknowledge Complexity: Meal planning doesn't have to be complicated. Start with some simple meals and gradually expand your repertoire.

Meal Planning for Special Diets

Whether you're vegetarian, vegan, gluten-free, or have other dietary restrictions, your meal plan can be customized to fit your specific needs. Here's how:

1. Recipe Research: Find recipes and resources that fit your dietary preferences and restrictions.

2. Substitutions: Learn how to substitute ingredients to adapt a recipe to your diet. For example, use gluten-free pasta and plant-based proteins.

3. Experiment: Don't be afraid to try new ingredients and flavors to fit your dietary needs.

Tools and Resources

Use these tools and resources to improve your meal planning:

1. Meal Planning Apps: Apps like Mealime, Plan to Eat and Paprika can help you organize recipes, create shopping lists, and plan meals efficiently.

2. Online recipe databases: Sites like Pinterest, Allrecipes, and Food Network offer a huge number of recipes to suit every taste and dietary preference.

3. Cookbooks: Expand your recipe repertoire by investing in cookbooks that focus on meal planning, quick meals, or specific cuisines.

4. Community Support: Join online meal planning forums and social media groups to exchange ideas, share recipes, and get support from like-minded people.

Conclusion

Mastering meal planning is a valuable skill that can simplify your life, improve your health, and save you time and money in the long run. Whether you're a beginner or an experienced meal planner, there's always room to hone your approach and discover new recipes and strategies. Start small and keep going to reap the benefits of stress-free, nutritious meals.

Meal planning isn't just a tedious task; it's a lifestyle choice that gives you control over your diet and overall health. Investing time and effort into meal planning will result in healthier habits, less stress, and more enjoyable meals to share with your loved ones. What are you waiting for? Start meal planning now and reap the benefits for years to come.

This comprehensive guide aims to help you understand the importance of meal planning and provide you with practical tips on how to effectively incorporate it into your daily life.

www.ingramcontent.com/pod-product-compliance
Lightning Source LLC
Chambersburg PA
CBHW070750250726
48662CB00004B/1734